Keto Bread:
Delicious Keto Bread Recipes Satisfy Your Bread Cravings, Burn Fat And Stay In Ketosis

By Sera Knight

COPY RIGHT STUFF

You May Also Like...

If you want to save time by bulk creating all your keto meals for the week all in one go, then this keto meal prep cookbook will help you do just that...

This keto meal prep cookbook will teach you how to successfully create many keto meals all in one go, and then store them so they remain fresh and actually taste nice when you reheat them.

Keto Meal Prep Cookbook: Save Time, Lose weight And Feel Great Throughout The Day.

Go Here To Find Out More...
https://www.amazon.com/dp/B07NJ85XMY

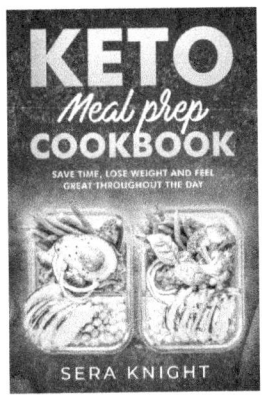

Get Your Free Keto Quick Start Guide Video...

Go To The Link Below To Gain Access To Your Free Keto Quick Start Guide Video...

https://ketodietexplorations.com/guide

Please Leave A Review

If you enjoy this **keto bread recipe book** and find it useful, then please would you be kind enough to leave it a review on Amazon.com

Go Here To Leave A Review For This Book On Amazon.com...

www.amazon.com/review/create-review?&asin=B07VJ8N78W

Thanks.

Sera Knight

Table Of Contents

What Is Keto Bread?

The rules for eating a keto diet are quite restrictive when it comes to bread. This is because a key part of the keto diet, is eating low amounts of carbs, and bread in general has a lot of carbs in it.

Get Your Free

Keto Quick Start Guide Video...

Go To The Link Below To Gain Access To Your Free Keto Quick Start Guide Video...

https://ketodietexplorations.com/guide

Traditionally made bread has too many carbs in it, to be a part of a keto diet. Luckily there are a number of low carb bread recipes that you can eat as a substitute .

It is possible for you to make your own low carb keto breads, using ingredients such as...

- Almond flour
- Coconut flour
- Psyllium husk
- Cream cheese
- Eggs

This book contains 21 of the best keto friendly breads, that you can make at home quickly and easily.

<u>Want To Know How To Make Keto Meals Faster?</u>

Go To The Link Below For A Keto Meal Prep System That Will Save You Hours Of Cooking Time Each Day...

https://www.amazon.com/dp/B07NJ85XMY

What Does Keto Mean?

A ketogenic or keto diet, involves eating low amounts of carbs. The reason for eating low amounts of carbs is because it can cause the body to burn more fat in a more efficient way.

Want To Know How To Make Keto Meals Faster?

Go To The Link Below For A Keto Meal Prep System That Will Save You Hours Of Cooking Time Each Day...

https://www.amazon.com/dp/B07NJ85XMY

How the keto diet got its name

As the glucose or sugar in your body are used up, your body will then switch over to burning stored fat as a fuel source instead.

When the body turns stored fat into fuel, it creates ketones. So the name keto actually comes from the first half of ketone.

To get your body to produce ketones, you can eat low amounts of carbs and a very small amount of protein. You need to eat lower protein, because your body is able to convert protein to blood sugar also.

A key role of your liver is to produce ketones from the stored fat on your body. Your body will only do this when there are no ready to access glucose in your blood stream.

The ketones that are produced by the liver, can then be used as a fuel source by your body and brain.

Your brain is able to run very well on both glucose or fat in the form of ketones.

Get Your Free Keto Quick Start Guide Video...

Go To The Link Below To Gain Access To Your Free Keto Quick Start Guide Video...

https://ketodietexplorations.com/guide

What Happens When A Person Goes Onto A Ketogenic Diet?

When a person goes onto a ketogenic diet, their body will switch over to using stored fat as a fuel source. This will help to burn off excess body fat faster.

Eating a keto diet has a number of health and weight loss benefits including...

- Reduced feelings of hunger

- Weight loss

- A more consistent stream of energy throughout the day, which will allow you to be more focused and alert throughout your day

- More steady blood sugar levels

- Higher levels of energy and mental clarity (less brain fog)

- Stomach feeling clearer

- Higher levels of physical endurance

- In certain cases, a keto diet can reduce the amount of seizures an epileptic has

Want To Know How To Make Keto Meals Faster?

Go To The Link Below For A Keto Meal Prep System That Will Save You Hours Of Cooking Time Each Day...

https://www.amazon.com/dp/B07NJ85XMY

As your body begins to produce ketones, it will go into a metabolic state that is called ketosis.

A very fast way to get into ketosis is through fasting. This involves not eating any food. The only problem with this is that no one can fast for ever.

You can instead eat a keto diet, and that will put you into and then keep you in that state known as ketosis.

Doing this will then give you many of the benefits of fasting, including weight loss, with out having to fast.

Get Your Free Keto Quick Start Guide Video...

Go To The Link Below To Gain Access To Your Free Keto Quick Start Guide Video...

https://ketodietexplorations.com/guide

Substitutes For Flour In Keto Baking

What are you trying to substitute for?

In normal full carb baking, the most important ingredients are...

- Gluten
- Starch

Gluten and starch are contained in the wheat flour used in the baking process.

Because you are baking keto bread, you will not be able to use wheat flour, and will need to add additional ingredients into your bread mixtures, that do similar jobs as gluten and starch.

What do gluten and starch do in the baking process...

Gluten

This is a type of protein in wheat flour. The gluten is responsible for the majority of the structure in bread baking or any other type of baking. High gluten flours also rise a lot higher, and brown more.

Starches

When you ferment bread, its the starch that gets eaten up by the yeast.

A big problem for keto baking, is that you can not use yeast in the baking process.

Because there is no food for the yeast to eat, there is nothing for it to ferment.

This means that you will not get a fluffy structure to your keto bread, that you would get in a yeast raised bread.

<u>The ingredients you can use in keto baking, to replicate the jobs that the starches and gluten found in wheat flour normly do...</u>

- Eggs
- Cream cheeses
- Psyllium husk fiber
- Almond flour
- Almond meal
- Coconut Flour
- Flex Meal
- Pumpkin Seed Meal

Eggs for keto baking

Eggs are great for making up for the lack of gluten in keto bread recipes. Gluten is one of the biggest contributors to the structure of non keto bread.

Eggs provide a lot of structure to keto bread, and can help to make up for the structure gluten would normally provide.

Eggs have great emulsifying properties, because of the egg yolk. This is good for keto bread baking because it helps to holed the batter or dough together. Also this will help to provide a bit more volume and texture to the keto breads you produce.

Cream cheeses for keto bread baking

This helps to add structure and chewiness to the keto breads you create.

Psyllium husk fiber for keto baking

Psyllium husk fiber can be used in keto breads where you want to get a more sourdough or rustic bread texture. Which can be difficult to achieve if you are using eggs as the main thickener or stabilizer of the bread.

Psyllium husk is made from the husk of the Psyllium seed, which has been ground down into a powder.

When water is added and mixed in with the Psyllium husk fiber, it will gel up , instead of simply absorbing the water. This then produces a gel like substance.

If you add enough water, and then heat it up, it will take on an extremely elastic structure, just like gluten.

What is psyllium husk?

Psyllium can be sold in either whole psyllium form or a psyllium powder.

The whole psyllium husks are more effective for baking. However, if you can only get the psyllium husk powder, then simply use it in an equal volume as you would for the recipe if its using he whole psyllium husk.

Psyllium husk powder or whole psyllium husk, can be used for gluten-free baking.

If you find it difficult to obtain psyllium husk at the shops, try looking in the health section.

Often it will be sold as a colon cleanser. This is because of its ability to absorb liquids.

You will be only using small amounts in the recipes so you will not be getting the full cleansing effect, unless you are consuming large amounts of bread made with psyllium husk in it.

Adding psyllium husk to your bread recipe will give your dough a thick, gooey consistency. This is the secret to greate gluten-free breads.

Almond flour for keto baking

What is almond flour?

Almond flour is made out of almonds. It is a gluten free nut flour, and consists of nothing but ground up blanched (without skin) almonds .

Almond flour is most often used as a low carb substitute for wheat flour, when making keto breads and other baked goods.

How to use almond flour?

Almond flour is a very common ingredient that can be used in many kinds of baked goods.

Because almonds do not contain gluten, any dough you create with almond flour will not behave like a traditional dough does.

A dough made with almond flour will not rise with yeast.

When you use almond flour in baking, you will need to add something to the recipe to absorb and bind the liquids.

The most common ingredients you can use for absorbing the liquids are...

- – Ground psyllium husk powder
- – Protein powder
- – And/or eggs

To know the number of grams of carbs per 100 grams of almond flour, check the label on the almond flour you buy.

Almond meal for keto baking

Almond meal can be created out of whole or blanched almonds. Almond flour has a consistency similar to corn meal as opposed to wheat flour.

Almond flour can be used in the baking of items for a low carbohydrate diet. Almond flour will add moistness and a nutty taste to bread and other baked goods.

Coconut Flour for keto baking

Coconut flour can be used as an alternative to wheat flour.

It can be used by those on a low carb diet or those who are intolerant to gluten.

There are several health benefits to eating coconut flour including...

- Stabilizing blood sugar
- Improved digestion
- Better heart health
- Weight loss

What is coconut flour?

Coconut flour is created out of coconut flesh, that is dried and ground up.

Coconut flour originated in the Philippines as a by-product of the creation of coconut milk.

To manufacture coconut flour, coconuts are first broken open and then drained of all liquids.

Then the coconut meat is scraped out. Then the coconut meat is rinsed, grated and strained in order to separate out the solids from the milk.

The solids are then baked at a very low temperature till they dry. Finally it is ground up into a flour.

The white coconut flour powder has a similar look to that of flour made from grains such as wheat. Coconut flour has a very mild coconut taste.

Coconut flour is a gluten free flour

Coconut flour is free from any gluten.

This makes coconut flour a good alternative for people who have

- Celiac disease
- Wheat allergy
- Non celiac gluten sensitivity

Benefits of eating coconut flour

Coconut flour can help to promote, stable blood sugar levels and also a healthier heart.

Additionally coconut flour can have antibacterial proprieties and may also aid digestion and weight loss.

Flex Meal for keto baking

Flex seeds are a very nutritious type of food.

One table spoon of whole flex seeds contains a high amount of healthy elements including...

- Omega-3 fatty acids
- Fiber
- Copper
- Magnesium
- Thiamin
- Manganese

Flex seeds that are ground up into flour are even more nutritionally dense. This is because they are in a easier form for your body to digest.

A great way to get more flax seed into your diet, is to use a flaxseed flour when you are creating baked goods.

Flax seed flour has a high concentration of oil, which means you can use it as a substitute for eggs or fat in some of the baked goods you produce.

Also flex seed flour is a good substitute for wheat flour.

You can use flex seed flour to create

- Breads
- Cookies
- Pancakes
- Cakes
- Muffins

Pumpkin Seed Meal for keto baking

Ground pumpkin seeds can add a gluten-free healthy boost to any keto bread you create.

Pumpkin seed meal is made out of ground up pumpkin seeds. Pumpkin seeds contain many health boosting ingredients and are a rich source of...

- Antioxidants

- Iron

- Zink

- Magnesium

Pumpkin seed meal when used to make bread, creates a great tasting and highly nutritious bread.

Low Carb Sweeteners You Can Use In Keto Baking

One of the main pillars of a ketogenic diet is to avoid almost all sugars and carbs.

Keeping your carbs macros super low, is what allows your body to trigger ketosis and start rapidly burning fat as an energy source.

Want To Know How To Make Keto Meals Faster?

Go To The Link Below For A Keto Meal Prep System That Will Save You Hours Of Cooking Time Each Day...

https://www.amazon.com/dp/B07NJ85XMY

For those who are new to a low carb diet, it can be tricky to fight the sugar cravings. However it is possible to overcome the sugar cravings, all it involves is 2 to 3 weeks of committing to staying off sugar entirely.

After you have weaned yourself off sugar entirely, you may find yourself with an urge for something sweet from time to time.

There are a number of ketogenic friendly sweeteners you can use to add the sweet taste into foods you create.

The top 3 ketogenic friendly sweeteners are...

1) Stevia

2) Erythritol

3) Xylitol

The best sweeteners for a keto diet

It is best to stick with stevia and erythritol, or a blend of the two.

Both are naturally occurring and don't cause blood sugar or insulin spikes, and they have a nice flavour.

Some people do complain of a slight after taste when they use stevia or erythritol on there own.

But when combined together the after tastes of each can be canceled out.

1) Stevia

Stevia comes from a herb which is more commonly known as the sugar leaf.

The extract version is nutrient free. Stevia has become popular with people on a keto diet, this is because it has sweet flavor, free from the detrimental effects of sugar.

Stevia sweeteners can come in a liquid or a crystal form, in many Supermarkets and natural food shops.

Studies on stevia have shown that stevia can reduce blood pressure, as well as lower blood glucose and insulin levels in diabetics.

Also animal testing of stevia, has shown that it has good results for producing anti-inflammatory effects.

Liquid stevia is raw powdered stevia, mixed with a solution that keeps it pure.

Powered stevia is often mixed with other sweeteners that can contain hidden carbs.

What is stevia exactly?

Stevia is a plant which is a member of the chrysanthemum family, and also a subgroup of the Asteraceae family (regweed family).

Stevia rebaudiana is the more official name for the plant.

The Stevia you can buy in shops is very different from the Stevia that you can grow yourself.

The Stevia sold in grocery stores, does not contain the whole of the Stevia leaf.

Instead they are made out of a highly refined Stevia leaf extract which is called rebaudioside A (Reb-A for short).

Rab-A is about 200 times more sweeter than sugar.

Rab-A can come in a number of forms including...
- Powder
- Liquid
- Granulated

What benefits are their to using Stevia?

Stevia is what is known as a non nutritive sweetener. This means that it contains almost no calories.

This can be useful if you are trying to lose weight.

If you have diabetes, Stevia can help to keep blood sugar levels stable.

How to use Stevia as a sugar replacement?

It is possible to use Stevia as a sugar replacement.

One pinch of Stevia powder is the equivalent of one teaspoon of sugar.

<u>Things Stevia can be added to include...</u>

- Tea and coffee

- Sprinkled on cereal

- Sprinkled on a unsweetened yogurt

- Put in smoothies

Stevia can be used in baking but may give the baked products a liquorice aftertaste.

Depending on the brand of Stevia you are using, you will have to play around with how much to use to achieve the desired tastes you prefer.

Because Stevia is so much more sweeter than sugar, you will need much less of it.

2) Erythritol

Erythritol is a sugar alcohol, that can naturally be found in fruits and vegetables. The commercial versions are normally extracted from corn.

Erythritol is an appropriate sweetener for a keto diet, this is because it doesn't affect blood sugar or insulin levels, and contains very few calories.

Erythritol is a low calorie sweetener. Some people say that Erythritol has all the good things about sugar without any of the negatives.

What is Erythritol?

Erythritol is what is known as a sugar alcohol.

Sugar alcohols are used by food producers to add a sweet flavour to the foods they produce.

Sugar alcohols have a molecular structure that allows them to stimulate the tongs sweet taste receptors.

3) Xylitol

Xylitol is also a sugar alcohol. Xylitol is not very nutrient dense and has a very similar taste to sugar.

Xylitol has also been found to help aid with dental health..

However, Xylitol has been closely linked to stomach discomfort in some people. And Xylitol is lethal for dogs.

Xylitol has a similar look and taste to sugar, but has less of the calories, and as a result will not raise blood sugar levels.

What is Xylitol?

Xylitol is what is known as a sugar alcohol.

Sugar alcohols have a chemical structure which allows them to stimulate the tongs taste receptors for sweetness in foods.

Xylitol can be found in tiny amounts in several fruits and vegetables, and is therefore classed as a natural sweetener.

The human body also produces small amounts as part of natural metabolism.

Xylitol is commonly used in things such as sugar free chewing gum, mints and diabetic friendly foods.

Xylitol is similar in sweetness to sugar but actually has 40 percent less calories. Xylitol from a shop will appear as a white crystalline powder, similar to sugar.

Because Xylitol is a refined sweetener, it contains no vitamins, minerals or proteins. Therefore it provides only empty calories.

Xylitol can be produced from the birch tree and similar trees, as well as from a plant fiber known as xylan.

Because sugar alcohols are carbohydrates, most of them actually do not raise blood sugar levels and as a result are not counted as net carbs, which makes them useful sweeteners for producing low-carb products such as keto bread.

The alcohols that are part of sugar alcohols are very different to those that get you drunk. Therefore they are safe for people who do not want to consume alcohol.

Xylitol for improved dental health

The bacteria in your mouth that cause plaque build-up and tooth decay, can not eat Xylitol and therefore will starve. This can therefore help to reduce cavities and inflammatory gums.

Summery of keto sweeteners

With any sweetener product that is labeled low or no carb, it is still important to look at the ingredients on the packaging.

Your goal should be to purchase the purest sweetener, and avoid products that contain fillers like...

- − Maltodextrin
- − Dextrose
- − Polydextrose

Because these can spike blood sugar and sometimes contain unnecessary carbs.

There are many products that claim to be sugar free, that actually contain ingredients that don't technically count as sugar, but still have a large glycemic index, such as Malatol.

<u>GI = Glycemic Index</u>

Each kind of sweetener usually contains some level of carbs and calories, and the ability to affect your blood sugar levels.

The Glycemic Index is a way to measuring how much a food will raise the blood sugar levels.

It is best to use sweeteners with the lowest GI.

Because of food labeling laws in the united states, a lot of products are permitted to calculate these additional ingredients out of the net carb counts, and can really add up as secret carbs.

Sweeteners to avoid when baking keto breads...

- Corn syrup
- White sugar
- Coconut sugar
- Fruit juice
- Maple syrup
- Honey
- Agave

Because they all contain very high levels of carbohydrates and high GI numbers and can spike the blood sugar levels and insulin.

<u>Want To Know How To Make Keto Meals Faster?</u>

Go To The Link Below For A Keto Meal Prep System That Will Save You Hours Of Cooking Time Each Day...

https://www.amazon.com/dp/B07NJ85XMY

Keto Bread Recipes...

This section of the book contains 20 delicious keto bread recipes.

Each recipe will tell you...

- How many servings it will produce

- Ingredients you will need

- Easy to follow step-by-step instructions for creating each of the keto bread recipes

Get Your Free Keto Quick Start Guide Video...

Go To The Link Below To Gain Access To Your Free Keto Quick Start Guide Video...

https://ketodietexplorations.com/guide

Keto Cloud Bread

Number Of Servings

- This recipe will make 6 servings

Ingredients needed...

- 3 ounces of mascarpon
- 1/8 a tea spoon of sea salt
- 3 large sized eggs (separate yolks and whites)
- (optional) 1/8 a tea spoon of cream of tartar

Preparation Instructions

1) Preheat your oven to 149 degrees C (300 degrees F)

2) Put into a large bowl the egg whites and cream of tartar, and beat with an electric mixer, until stiff peaks begin to form.

3) Next in a second large sized bowl, place the egg yolks, mascarpone, and the sea salt, and mix together until the mixture is smooth.

4) Next fold the egg whites mixture in with the mascarpone mixture, using a spatula. As you are folding the two mixtures together, ensure you don't brake down the air bubbles in the egg whites.

5) Next, line a baking tray with some parchment paper, and then grease the paper lightly.

6) Now scoop the mixture, into 6 circular discs on the parchment paper.

7) Bake for 25 to 35 minutes, or until golden.

Keto Flaxseed Bread

Number Of Servings

- This recipe will produce 10 servings

Ingredients needed...

- 5 eggs
- 1 table spoon of dried oregano
- 1 tea spoon of pink salt
- 2 cups of flax seed meal
- 1/3 a cup of avocado oil
- ½ a cup of water
- 1 table spoon of baking powder (gluten free)

Preparation Instructions

1) Preheat your oven to 350 F.

2) Line a 13 X 9 baking pan with parchment paper

3) Put the dry ingredients into a mixing bowl: baking powder, salt, flaxseed meal, oregano. Put to one side.

4) Put into the blender the eggs and the oil. And then blend for 30 seconds, until the mixture becomes frothy.

5) Pour the egg mixture into the bowl of the dry ingredients, and mix together well with a spatula. Also add the water and mix well. Allow this mixture to sit for about 5 minutes.

6) Pour the mixture into the baking pan that's been lined with baking paper.

7) Put into the oven for 20 minutes, or until the top becomes firm and golden.

8) Remove from oven, and allow to cool on a cooling rack.

9) Cut up the bread into 10 pieces, and enjoy

Additional Notes....

- You can keep this bread in the fridge for up to 4 days.
- This bread is freezer friendly, and tastes great when toasted and buttered.

Get Your Free Keto Quick Start Guide Video...

Go To The Link Below To Gain Access To Your Free Keto Quick Start Guide Video...

https://ketodietexplorations.com/guide

Keto Poppy Seed Bread

Number Of Servings

- This recipe will produce 8 servings

Ingredients needed...

- 3 eggs
- 4 table spoons of chia seeds (or flax seed)
- 1 tea spoon of baking powder
- 1 tea spoon of salt
- 8 ounces of cottage cheese
- 1 table spoon of olive oil
- 4 table spoons of sun flour seeds
- 1 tea spoon of ground psyllium husk (powder)
- 1 table spoon of poppy seeds

Preparation Instructions

1) Put all the dry ingredients into a bowl and mix up well.

2) Now stir in to this mixture the eggs, oil, and cottage cheese, and mix together evenly.

3) Allow this mixture to sit for 15 minutes

4) Line a baking sheet with parchment paper.

5) Spread the mixture out of the bowl, onto the parchment lined baking sheet.

6) Bake in a preheated oven at 175 C (350 F) for 20 to 25 minutes.

7) Once baked, place onto a rack to dry. (without parchment paper)

8) Once dry, cut up into 8 servings, and add butter and any other desired toppings.

<u>Additional notes...</u>

- You can store in fridge for 4 days

- Freeze if you want to store for longer

- This bread tastes amazing toasted right out of the freezer with a little butter.

<u>Want To Know How To Make Keto Meals Faster?</u>

Go To The Link Below For A Keto Meal Prep System That Will Save You Hours Of Cooking Time Each Day...

https://www.amazon.com/dp/B07NJ85XMY

Keto Onion Bread

<u>Number Of Servings</u>

- This recipe will produce 15 slices of bread

<u>Ingredients needed...</u>

- 5 table spoons of coconut oil
- 1 table spoon of erythritol
- ½ tea spoon of sea salt
- ¾ a cup of coconut flour (that has been sifted)
- 6 large sized eggs
- ¼ a cup of (unsweetened) coconut milk
- 3 table spoons of organic onion flakes
- 1 tea spoon of baking powder

Preparation Instructions

1) Pre heat your oven to 175 C (350 F)

2) Brake the 5 eggs into a mixing bowl, and slightly beat them.

3) Add to the eggs in the mixing bowl, the coconut oil, coconut milk, onion flakes, lachanto, salt, and baking powder. And whisk all these ingredients together well.

4) Now add the coconut flour to this mixture.

5) Now, grease a loaf pan (sized 9x5x3 inch)

6) Pour the mixture into the greased loaf pan.

7) Bake the mixture for 40 to 45 minutes at 175 C (350 F)

8) Once baked, remove from the oven and allow to cool for 10 to 15 minutes. (before removing from the loaf pan)

9) Cut slices when you need them

Keto Cheese And Onion Bread

Number Of Servings

- This recipe will produce 8 servings.

Ingredients needed...

- ½ tea spoon of yeast
- 2 whole eggs
- 3/4 a cup of only egg whites
- 2 table spoons of (grated) parmesan cheese
- Toppings (of your choice)
- 1 cup of shredded cheddar cheese
- 4 table spoons of warm water
- 1 cup of trim healthy mama baking blend
- 2 tea spoons of baking soda
- ½ a tea spoon of Italian seasoning
- ¼ a medium red onion, sliced into one inch pieces and sautéed

Preparation Instructions

1) Add to the warm water, the yeast and stir. Allow to sit as you prepare the rest of the recipe.

2) In a 8 inch skillet (that will fit into your oven) sauté the onions.

3) Put the sautéed onions in a bowl, and sit to one side for now.

4) Now in a large mixing bowl, mix together all the remaining ingredients. And allow to sit for 5 minutes. (this allows it time to thicken slightly)

5) Pour the batter into the pan and sprinkle with the onion and cheese.

6) Use your finger, to dimple the top of the batter slightly.

7) Sprinkle on any other seasoning.

8) Bake at 350 F (175 C) for about 30 minutes (until the top goes a light brown)

9) Remove from the oven, and allow to cool for 15 minutes.

<u>Want To Know How To Make Keto Meals Faster?</u>

Go To The Link Below For A Keto Meal Prep System That Will Save You Hours Of Cooking Time Each Day...

https://www.amazon.com/dp/B07NJ85XMY

Keto Flatbread

- This recipe will create one loaf of bread

Ingredients needed...

- 1 cup (100 g) of mozzarella cheese (shredded)
- 1 large sized egg (beaten)
- 2 (minced) cloves of garlic
- ½ a tea spoon of dried thyme
- 1 table spoon of cream cheese
- ¼ a cup (30 g) of almond flour
- ½ a tea spoon of dried oregano
- 1 tea spoon of fresh rosemary (minced)
- add salt and pepper to taste

Preparation Instructions

1) Combine in a medium sized bowl the mozzarella and cream cheese.

2) Microwave this mixture in 30 second intervals, stirring between each microwave session, until the cheese has fully melted and has formed a smooth consistency. (normally takes about one minute overall)

3) Allow the cheese to cool for a few minutes (to prevent the eggs from scrambling in the next step)

4) Now add to the bowl the egg, garlic, thyme, salt, pepper, almond flour, oregano, rosemary. And stir until well combined.

5) Pre heat your oven to 180 C (350 F).

6) While you wait for the oven to pre heat, line a baking tray with parchment paper.

7) Pour the mixture onto the baking tray, and flatten out into an even layer about ½ an inch thick.

8) Now bake for about 10 to 15 minutes, until the bread turns a golden brown.

9) You can serve this bread in a number of ways including, sliced into chips, cut up into bread sticks, top with a source and toppings of your choice, or use to create a pizza.

Get Your Free Keto Quick Start Guide Video...

Go To The Link Below To Gain Access To Your Free Keto Quick Start Guide Video...

https://ketodietexplorations.com/guide

Keto Flatbread Matzo

<u>Number Of Servings</u>

- This will create one flat bread.

<u>Ingredients needed...</u>

- 3 table spoons of unsalted butter (cold)
- 2 table spoons of (ground) sage
- 2 tea spoons of salt
- ¼ a cup of almond flour
- 4 large sized eggs
- 3 table spoons of onion powder

Preparation Instructions

1) Pre heat your oven to 350 F

2) Separate the egg whites from the yolks

3) Whip the egg whites until they forms stiff peaks.

4) Mix to the whipped egg whites, the spices and half of the almond flour.

5) Add next, the butter (cut into bits), the egg yolks, and the other half of the almond flour. And mix together.

6) Spread the mixture on a baking tray, that has had parchment paper placed on it.

7) Bake for 10 – 12 minutes, at 350 F.

8) Then increase the heat to 400 F and cook for 4 to 5 more minutes.

9) Remove from oven, allow to cool.

10) Cut up into 8 pieces ready to serve.

__Keto Pita Bread__

<u>Number Of Servings</u>

- This recipe will produce 12 servings

<u>Ingredients needed...</u>

- ½ a cup (100 g) of almond flour
- 4 table spoons of coconut flour
- 1 table spoon of sesame seeds
- ½ a tea spoon of sea salt
- 1/3 a cup (60 g) of butter
- 50 ml of water (optional)
- 2 table spoons of psyllium powder
- 4 table spoons of flaxseed flour
- 1 tea spoon of dried rosemary (chopped or ground)
- 2 large sized eggs
- 4 table spoons of olive oil (extra virgin)

Preparation Instructions

1) Put all the dry ingredients in to a large sized mixing bowl, and mix all the dry ingredients together well.

2) In a pan melt the butter and mix in the olive oil.

3) Add the eggs to the pan and beat into the butter and oil, using a whisk.

4) Combine the dry and wet ingredients together in the mixing bowl. Then work into a dough with your hands. (add sprinkles of water if the dough is too dry).

5) Next, put the dough into the freezer for about 10 minutes.

6) Next, brake off balls of dough, big enough to roll between two sheets of parchment paper, and turn into 5mm thick pita bread pieces.

7) Grill the pita bread (1 – 2 minutes each side)

8) If you would like crunchy pita bread, then grill for about 4 minutes (make sure not to grill too long to prevent burning).

Keto Naan Bread And Melted Garlic Butter

<u>Number Of Servings</u>

- This recipe will make 8 servings

<u>Ingredients needed...</u>

- 4 ounces of butter
- 2 minced garlic cloves
- 2 table spoons of ground psyllium husk powder
- ½ a tea spoon of baking powder
- 1/3 a cup of melted coconut oil
- coconut oil, Optional) for frying
- ¾ a cup of coconut flour
- ½ a tea spoon of onion powder (optional)
- 1 tea spoon of salt
- 2 cups of water (boiling)
- sea salt

Preparation Instructions

1) Put all the dry ingredients into a bowl, and mix well.

2) Now add to the mixture the oil and boiling water, and stir together well.

3) Allow the mixture to rise for 5 minutes.

4) The dough should turn firm very fast, and remain flexible.

If you have got the mixture right, the dough will resemble the consistency of play doh.

If the dough is too runny,, then add extra psyllium husk , until it has the right feel.

If the dough is too firm, then add some additional water.

5) Split the dough up into 6 to 8 even pieces.

6) Turn each piece of dough into a ball, and then flatten out with your hands on a piece of parchment paper.

7) Fry the nann in a skillet, over a medium heat, to the point when the naan turns a nice golden color.(add coconut oil so the naan bread doesn't stick)

8) In a pan, melt the butter, and add the freshly squeeze garlic.

9) Use a brush to apply the melted butter to the bread pieces, and lightly sprinkle the top with salt.

 10) Pour the remaining garlic butter into a bowl, and dip bits of the bread into it.

Want To Know How To Make Keto Meals Faster?

Go To The Link Below For A Keto Meal Prep System That Will Save You Hours Of Cooking Time Each Day...

https://www.amazon.com/dp/B07NJ85XMY

Keto Poori Bread

Number Of Servings

- This recipe produces 6 servings

Ingredients needed...

- 1 cup of thick mozzarella (shredded)
- ¼ a tea spoon of baking powder
- 1 table spoon of almond flour (back up)
- ½ a cup of almond flour
- 1 ounce of cream cheese
- 1 egg

Reparation Instructions

1) Put into a mixing bowl the almond flour and the baking powder and mix well.

2) Next, add the mozzarella and cream cheese to the bowl also. And microwave the mixture for 1 minute (in 30 second intervals)

3) Now add the eggs and use a spatula to mix the melted mozzarella in with the other ingredients. (before it cools down too much)

4) If the dough is too wet, add one table spoon of almond flour.

5) Roll the dough out between two sheets of parchment paper. (to about ¼ an inch thickness)

6) Next, use a ramekin (or small bowl) to cut the dough out into round pieces.

7) Lightly dust each round with a little bit of the almond flour.

8) Heat the oil of your choice in a frying pan

9) Test your oil temperature is ready, by dropping a small piece of the dough into the pan. When it sizzles and rises to the top of the oil, it is hot enough to use)

10) Now, drop a dough round (one at a time, into the oil in the pan. It should now rise to the top of the oil.

11) Now use a slotted spoon, to spoon some of the oil on to the top of the Poori, and make sure the bottom is not over cooked.

12) When the Poori puffs up and goes a golden brown, flip it over and allow the other side to brown also.

13) Once both sides are a light golden brown, then remove them from the oil using the slotted spoon. And place them on a paper towel.

14) Allow to cool slightly, but serve warm for best taste.

<u>Want To Know How To Make Keto Meals Faster?</u>

Go To The Link Below For A Keto Meal Prep System That Will Save You Hours Of Cooking Time Each Day...

https://www.amazon.com/dp/B07NJ85XMY

Keto Soft Seed Bread

Number Of Servings

- This recipe will produce 20 servings.

Ingredients needed...

- ¾ a cup of coconut flour
- ½ a cup of flaxseed
- 3 tea spoons of baking powder
- 1 tea spoon of salt
- 7 ounces of cream cheese
- ¾ a cup of whipping cream (heavy)
- 1 cup of almond flour
- 5 and 1/3 a table spoon of sesame seeds
- ¼ a cup of ground psyllium husk (powder)
- 1 tea spoon of ground caraway seeds (or fennel seeds)
- 6 eggs
- ½ a cup of melted coconut oil (or butter)
- 1 table spoon of poppy (or sesame) seeds

Preparation Instructions

1) Remove the cream cheese from the fridge, and allow to come to room temperature. (so it will blend better)

2) Pre heat your oven to 175 C (350 F)

3) Put all the dry ingredients, (except for the poppy or sesame seeds, which will be used for topping the bread) into a mixing bowl. And mix together evenly.

4) In a second mixing bowl put all the remaining ingredients, and whisk until they form a smooth consistency.

5) Next, add the dry mix of ingredients in with the batter mix, and mix together well.

6) Now, place the dough into a greased bread pan. (4 x 7 inches).

7) Bake the bread for about 45 minutes, on the lowest shelf in the oven.

8) To know when fully cooked, prick the bread with a knife, when it comes out clean, it is done.

9) Remove from the oven and remove from the pan.

10) Remove the parchment paper, place on a rack and allow to cool.

11) Slice and add your favorite toppings.

Get Your Free Keto Quick Start Guide Video...

Go To The Link Below To Gain Access To Your Free Keto Quick Start Guide Video...

https://ketodietexplorations.com/guide

Keto Coconut Flour Bread

Number Of Servings

-   This recipe will produce 14 servings.

Ingredients needed...

-   1/3 a cup of olive oil (or coconut oil) (or butter)
-   ½ a cup of coconut flour
-   2 table spoons of erythritol
-   1 tea spoon of xanthan gum
-   1 tea spoon of ground cinnamon
-   6 eggs
-   1/3 a cup of water (or a heavy cream) (or coconut milk)
-   ½ a cup of ground flax seed
-   1 table spoon of baking powder
-   ½ a tea spoon of salt

Preparation Instructions

1) Pre heat your oven to 375 F

2) Place into a food mixer (or blender) the eggs, milk or cream, oil and blend up until well combined.

3) Next, add the remaining ingredients to the blender, and mix together also.

4) Sprinkle the toasted sesame seeds on top of the loaf (if you desire).

5) Next, line a 8 x 4 loaf pan, with parchment paper.

6) Pour the batter into the loaf pan.

7) Bake for about 40 to 45 minutes, until a knife pricked in will come out clean)

8) Remove from oven and allow to cool on rack for 20 minutes.

9) Allow to cool completely before slicing.

10) Add toppings of your choice to each slice.

Keto Almond Flour Bread

Number Of Servings

- This recipe will produce 12 servings.

Ingredients needed...

- 2 egg whites
- 2 eggs
- ¼ a cup of butter (60 g) (melted)
- 1 and ½ a tea spoon of baking powder
- A pinch of salt
- 2 cups of almond flour (200 g)
- 4 table spoons of psyllium husk
- ½ a tea spoon of xanthan gum
- ½ a cup of warm water

Preparation Instructions

1) Pre heat your oven to 180 C (350 F)

2) Put 2 eggs and the egg whites from two eggs in a mixing bowl, and beat together (use the two remaining eggs to create mayonnaise if you desire).

3) Add the remaining ingredients into a mixing bowl also, and blend until you have a smooth dough. Be careful not to over mix.

4) Pour dough into a small loaf pan (7 x 4 inches).

5) Bake for 45 minutes (until you can prick with knife and it comes out clean.)

Want To Know How To Make Keto Meals Faster?

Go To The Link Below For A Keto Meal Prep System That Will Save You Hours Of Cooking Time Each Day...

https://www.amazon.com/dp/B07NJ85XMY

Keto Savory Bread

Number Of Servings

- This recipe will produce about 3 medium sized loaves.
- 12 slices per loaf
- 36 slices in total

Ingredients needed...

- ¼ a cup of coconut flour
- 8 ounces of cream cheese
- 1 tea spoon of rosemary seasoning
- 2 table spoons of parsley seasoning
- 2 and ½ cups of almond flour
- ½ a cup of butter
- 8 whole eggs
- 1 tea spoon of sage seasoning
- 1 and ½ a tea spoon of baking powder

Preparation Instructions

1) Place into a medium sized mixing bowl, the butter and cream cheese, until it forms a smooth consistency.

2) Next, add to the mixture the sage, parsley seasoning, and whisk until fully mix together well.

3) Next add the eggs, and mix in also.

4) Now, add the flour and baking powder. And mix in also.

5) Next, grease 3 mid sized loaf pans.

6) Then, fill each loaf pan about half way with the batter.

7) Bake the bread for about 35 minutes, at 350 F.

8) When cooked well, it will have a golden brown colour on top, and a knife pricked into the bread will come out clean.

9) Remove from oven and allow to cool.

10) Remove from loaf pans.

11) Slice and add your toppings of choice. (each loaf will procure 12 slices, depending on how thinly or thickly you slice your bread)

<u>Get Your Free Keto Quick Start Guide Video...</u>

Go To The Link Below To Gain Access To Your Free Keto Quick Start Guide Video...

https://ketodietexplorations.com/guide

Keto Pumpkin Bread

- This recipe will produce 12 servings.

Ingredients needed...

- ½ a cup of coconut flour
- 2 tea spoons of pumpkin pie spice
- ¼ a sea spoon of sea salt
- 4 large eggs
- ¼ a cup of pumpkin seeds
- 2 cups of blanched almond flour
- ¾ a cup of erythritol
- 2 tea spoons of baking powder
- ¾ a cup of pumpkin puree
- 1/3 a cup of butter

Preparation Instructions

1) Pre heat your oven to 177 C (350 F)

2) Line a 9 x 5 inch loaf pan, with parchment paper.

3) Place into a large mixing bowl, the almond flour, erythritol, baking powder, coconut flour, pumpkin pie spice, sea salt. Mix all these ingredients together well.

4) Next, add to this mix, the pumpkin puree, eggs and the butter (melted). Mix all ingredients together well.

5) Pour the batter into the lined loaf pan.

6) Press down on the top of the batter to give it a smooth top.

7) Sprinkle the pumpkin seeds on the top of the loaf, and press in lightly.

8) Bake for 50 to 60 minutes.

9) When you can prick the loaf with a knife and it comes out clean, then it has finished baking.

10) Remove from the oven and place on rack and allow to cool completely before removing from the pan and slicing.

11) Add your favourite toppings to a slice and enjoy.

Keto Cauliflower Bread

Number Of Servings

- This recipe will produce one loaf of cauliflower bread.

Ingredients needed...

- ¼ a cup of psyllium husk
- ½ a tea spoon of baking soda
- 5 eggs (beaten)
- 2 cups of almond flour
- ½ a tea spoon of salt
- 1 cup of steamed cauliflower rice
- cooking spray

Ingredients for decoration...

- 1 tea spoon of pumpkin seeds
- 1 tea spoon of sun flower seeds
- 1 tea spoon of sesame seeds

Preparation Instructions

1) Preheat your oven to 350 F

2) Spray the sides and bottom of loaf pan with cooking spray.

3) Line the loaf pan with parchment paper.

4) Prepare the cauliflower rice (see later instructions)

5) Place into a large mixing bowl, the almond flour, salt, psyllium husk, and baking soda. And mix together well.

6) Next, fold the eggs and the cauliflower into the mixture. Mix the batter until it becomes smooth.

7) Pour the batter into the loaf pan and use a spatula to smooth out on top.

8) Sprinkle the top of the loaf with the sunflower seeds, pumpkin seeds, and the sesame seeds. Press down lightly into the loaf.

9) Bake the loaf for about 55 minutes, until the top of the bread becomes a golden brown.

10) Test the loaf is cooked properly, by piercing with a knife and when it comes out clean, its cooked well throughout.

11) When finished cooking, remove from the oven and allow to cool before removing from pan and slicing.

12) Slice and add toppings of your choice.

Want To Know How To Make Keto Meals Faster?

Go To The Link Below For A Keto Meal Prep System That Will Save You Hours Of Cooking Time Each Day...

https://www.amazon.com/dp/B07NJ85XMY

Instructions for creating cauliflower rice...

1) Wash the cauliflower thoroughly.

2) Remove any greens from the cauliflower, and cut up into 4 equal pieces.

3) Use the medium sized holes on a grater, to grate the cauliflower into rice like pieces. (leave any large tough bits out)

4) Place the cauliflower rice pieces into a clean bowl.

5) Use a paper towel to press on the cauliflower rice, to remove any excess moisture.

6) Next, sauté the cauliflower rice , in a large skillet, on a medium heat, in one table spoon of olive oil. Cook but do not brown, until the cauliflower rice becomes tender. (about 5 to 8 minutes)

7) Use this cauliflower rice in the recipe as instructed above.

Keto Walnut And Zucchini Bread

<u>Number Of Servings</u>

- This recipe will produce one loaf

<u>Ingredients needed...</u>

- ½ a cup of butter
- 1 zucchini (grated)
- ½ a tea spoon of salt
- ½ a cup of coconut flour
- 6 eggs
- ½ a cup of walnuts (that have been coarsely chopped)
- 1 tea spoon of xantham gum

Preparation Instructions

1) Into a large mixing bowl, grate the zucchini.

2) Place all the other ingredients (except the walnuts) into the mixing bowl also. And mix with an electric mixer for 1 to 2 minutes.

3) Grease a loaf tray.

4) Put the ingredients into the loaf tray.

5) Level out the top of the loaf and place the walnuts evenly on the top of the loaf.

6) Bake for about 50 minutes at 180 C (350 F)

7) Remove from oven and allow to cool.

8) Once cooled remove from pan and slice.

9) Add toppings of your choice to a slice and enjoy.

Keto Coconut Flour Bread In A Mug

Number Of Servings

- This recipe will produce one serving

Ingredients needed...

- 1 table spoon of heavy whipping cream
- 1 egg
- salt to taste
- 2 table spoons of coconut flour
- 1 table spoon of olive oil
- ¼ tea spoon of baking powder

Preparation Instructions

1) Put all ingredients into a mixing bowl, and mix together well.

2) Pour into mug (mix all ingredients in mug to cut down on washing up).

3) Microwave for 90 seconds.

4) Remove from microwave and remove from mug.

5) Slice.

6) Add toppings of your choice and enjoy.

Get Your Free Keto Quick Start Guide Video...

Go To The Link Below To Gain Access To Your Free Keto Quick Start Guide Video...

https://ketodietexplorations.com/guide

Keto Almond Flour Blueberry Muffins

Number Of Servings

- This recipe will produce 12 muffins.

Ingredients needed...

- ½ a cup of erythritol
- ¼ a tea spoon of sea salt
- 1/3 a cup of unsweetened almond milk
- ½ a tea spoon of vanilla extract
- 2 and ½ a cup of blanched almond flour
- 1 and ½ a tea spoon of gluten free baking powder#
- 1/3 a cup of coconut oil
- 3 large eggs
- ¾ a cup of blueberries

Preparation Instructions

1) Pre heat your oven to 177C (350F).

2) Next, Line a muffin pan with 12 parchment paper muffin liners.

3) Put into a large mixing bowl, the almond flour, baking powder, erythritol and sea salt. And stir together well.

4) Next, add to the mixture the coconut oil (melted), almond milk, vanilla extract and eggs. Mix together well.

5) Next, add the blueberries to the mixture, and fold in to the mixture.

6) Place an even amount of the batter into each of the 12 muffin cups.

7) Bake the muffins for about 20 to 25 minutes, until their tops become golden, and a knife piercing a muffin comes out clean

8) Remove from oven and allow to cool on a rack.

9) Eat and enjoy.

<u>Want To Know How To Make Keto Meals Faster?</u>

Go To The Link Below For A Keto Meal Prep System That Will Save You Hours Of Cooking Time Each Day...

https://www.amazon.com/dp/B07NJ85XMY

Keto Avocado Cloud Bread

Number Of Servings

- This recipe will produce 12 servings.

Ingredients needed...

- ¼ a tea spoon of cream of tartar
- a pinch of salt
- 4 eggs (separated)
- ½ a ripe avocado (mashed up)
- 2 tea spoons of toasted sesame seeds

Preparation Instructions

1) Pre heat your oven to 300 F.

2) Line a large sized baking tray with parchment paper.

3) Put into a large mixing bowl the egg whites and cream of tartar, and use a hand mixer to beat this mixture until it forms stiff peaks.

4) Place into a medium sized mixing bowl, the avocado, egg yolks and salt.

5) Use a hand mixer to mix these ingredients together until smooth.

6) Next fold in the egg whites mixture from the other bowl, until smooth and mixed well.

7) Use about ¼ a cup of the dough to create round and flattened pieces of bread. Spread out about an inche aparte on the baking tray.

8) Sprinkle each piece of bread with sesame seeds.

9) Bake for about 30 to 35 minutes, until golden and firm.

10) Remove from oven, and allow to cool.

11) Add toppings of your choice and enjoy.

<u>Get Your Free Keto Quick Start Guide Video...</u>

Go To The Link Below To Gain Access To Your Free Keto Quick Start Guide Video...

https://ketodietexplorations.com/guide

You May Also Like...

If you want to save time by bulk creating all your keto meals for the week all in one go, then this keto meal prep cookbook will help you do just that...

This keto meal prep cookbook will teach you how to successfully create many keto meals all in one go, and then store them so they remain fresh and actually taste nice when you reheat them.

Keto Meal Prep Cookbook:

Save Time, Lose weight And Feel Great Throughout The Day.

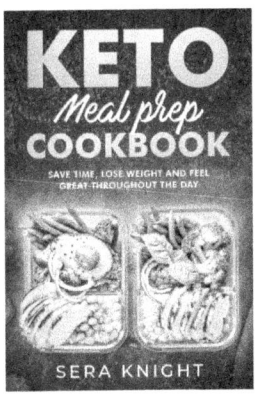

Go Here To Find Out More...
https://www.amazon.com/dp/B07NJ85XMY

Get Your Free Keto Quick Start Guide Video...

Go To The Link Below To Gain Access To Your Free Keto Quick Start Guide Video...

https://ketodietexplorations.com/guide

Thank You

It has been a real pleasure putting all of these keto bread recipes together for you in this book.

I am truly thankful you purchased this book.

Thank you for downloading and reading this book right to the end.

If you enjoyed this book and found it useful then...

Please leave your review of this book on Amazon...

Go Here To Leave A Review For This Book On Amazon.com...

www.amazon.com/review/create-review?&asin=B07VJ8N78W

Thanks again.

Sera Knight